I0423382

Eating Clean But Keep It Lean

Weight Loss Secrets and Recipes – Soups and Salads

Healthy Cooking made easy with American and European (metric and imperial) measures. Calorie, Fat, Protein and Carb calculations for every recipe

Cook and eat at home or brown bag it for lunch.

Maia Lloyd

Three Peas Publishing

First Edition

"Eating Clean But Keep It Lean" Series

DISCLAIMER

Introduction

What you will gain from this book:

1. The **knowledge to make your clean eating and weight loss efforts a success, based on my expertise as a nutritionist with five weight loss clinics** in London;
2. Simple, delicious recipes that are **tried and tested in my weight loss clinics** to help you get and stay lean. **Recogisable, good food. No weird ingredients you have to Google to find out what they are**.; and
3. **Encouragement to commit to this supportive, sustainable way o**f eating. No three juices a day and starvation. Real, nutritious food to help you look great, prevent disease and age well.

It works for my clients and it can work for you.

This series is called "Eating Clean But Keep It Lean" because my approach is clean eating (which I will explain). I focus on dropping weight as part of a clean diet so I will support your healthy aims and help you identify the elements of clean eating that may be holding your weight loss back.

My recipes are deliberately simple so you can use them every day. No long ingredients lists or complicated food prep.

This book is about Soups and Salads.

To give you a flavour (lot's, actually) of the recipes in the second half of this book, we have:

- A clean and lean **Caesar Salad**. Yes, that favourite but leaned up so you can eat it and lose weight
- **Chinese chicken, green mango and mint salad**. You can also serve this one hot and ot would make a great summer supper or for entertaining. I am about food that does not ake you a freak and I expect you to be doing more with life as you adopt my programme, not hiding under a duvet for the rest of your life.
- **Turkey and brocolli salad with gremolata**. Gremolata is just a posh name for a citrusy, herby dressing. The turkey in this recipe contains tryptophan, which keeps you calm and centred. The broccoli helps your liver detox and as a result, gives your skin that glows. *That's a much better look than sad and starving, don't you think?*
- **Courgette and white bean soup**. Imagine having a bowl of this handmade soup (don't worry, it only takes 5 minutes to make – literally) for lunch. How much better than a shop bought sandwich in a packet.
- **Mexican pinto bean soup with avocado salsa**. If you take this one to work, your colleagues will be jealous! You could also have this with friends on a night in and show them what Eating Clean But Keep It Lean looks and tastes like.

So, the recipes sound pretty good, don't they? The nutrition behind it is planned by me, a nutritionist and weight loss speciaist. At my clinics, I do weight loss and nothing else so I do know what I am talking about and I am paid to help clients get results.

Let me help you. So let's go!

Why is eating clean the right starting point?

You want to eat clean _and_ lose weight? Clean does not always mean lean – all that brown rice syrup and gluten fee flour is high carb and will not drop the pounds.

This book will fit your clean nutritional goals _and_ get you in shape.

Lunch is the least planned meal of the day – grab something on the go, buy a sandwich or a pre-packed soup or salad. But what is in it? Is it really clean? If it is, what's the price premium? Make your own lunches which mean you are Eat Clean But Keep It Lean every day, and you save money

If you are thinking about trying the clean approach, what you will you gain from being a bit more thoughtful about what you eat? Is it all hype?

As a nutritonal therapist with five clinics that I run for weightloss and health, I can sat categorically, that it is not all hype:

If you are tired of feeling tired; or

You want that glow in your skin, hair and eyes that says that you are confident in your own skin and you eat right; or

You want your complexion and your skin tone to age gently not crash into sags and wrinkles (I kid you not).

Eating clean will help you.

It is like putting in natural fertiliser with your watering system for your plants. Look at the difference you see in plants that are getting the super boost of nutrients – glossy leaves, bigger plants, more flowers, more intense colours.

Eating clean is about eating nutrient dense meals so you soup (no pun intended) up your nutrition: you get the natural fertiliser, if you will.

So this book, and the rest of my "Eating Clean But Keep it Lean" series, provides nutritionally analysed and calorie, fat, protein and carbohydrate assessed recipes that do the following for you:

(1) push health-giving nutrients into your cells; and

(2) eat clean but lean so if you have any excess weight to shift, it shifts quickly enough for you to see results and you stay motivated.

Why lunch is important

Some of you reading this will probably understand only too well, how important lunch, or any meal, is. At my clinics when I work one to one with clients, we are often talking about dialing back the importance of food beyond pleasure in the moment and towardsgood nutrition for your body, long term.

But you might be in the other camp: dieters who skips meals to manage calories. You might be thinking – why not skip lunch, save the calories?

That is like the modern equivalent of the famous line from the movie Wall Street – "Lunch is for wimps!'

Well, lunch is not for wimps, it is for the smart. Your body needs to be fed with nutrients for it to function, including brain function and fat loss. If you want to do more than just get through the day, you need to feel great with steady energy levels. If you skip lunch, your blood sugar will be high and then low: the same will be the case with your energy levels.

Second, skipping lunch also causes an energy, hormone and mood rollercoaster that causes over-eating, unhealthy snacking and bingeing later in the day. Quite apart from what the snacks are doing to your body, you will feel terrible: emotionally raw, overwhelmed and tired.

If you skip lunch, your body goes into famine mode and you will start breaking down muscle for energy. You need muscle to feel well and be able to handle your day. Muscle is also the engine that burns energy and calories, so if you burn muscle, you depress your metabolism, making it easier to gain weight.

Third, your body slows down lots of processes in response to nutritional famine, particularly hormone production. So skipping lunch can make you *feel* low, have low sex drive and even have difficulty getting pregnant.

So what about having lunch but just something small? Well it depends what you choose. Grabbing the wrong lunch is almost as bad. That slice of pizza or deli noodle salad might look small but it will fail the clean but lean test. It will be full of unhealthy fats and sugars. It may also have all sorts of hidden nasties like artificial additives. A lunch loaded with not so clean ingredients – processed, preserved and generally foods not in their natural state.

A clean eating lunch is one that silences hunger pangs and nourishes your body. It should carry you through to an afternoon snack and then dinner free from sugar or salt cravings. Eat clean at lunch and your brain will feel focused and your body energetic.

Sounds too good to be true, right? Wrong.

These lunch recipes with their focus on clean but lean will keep your energy levels up to support you so you are able to bound around all day. Your body will be firing out signals to build up, not break down, so your muscles will be building and building your metabolism. Your mood will be supported so you end up with a virtuous circle: look after yourself nutritionally = body functioning optimally to support your metabolism and your organs, including skin and hair; a decrease in body fat due to overall healthy balance of clean but lean eating is trhe result.

First some basics on clean eating (If you've read my Breakfast book in this programme, you can skip straight to the next chapter).

The basics of a clean programme

Let's talk about what clean eating entails: eating clean means eating whole foods, in as natural a state as possible. It can include raw foods or vegetarian or vegan dishes. But equally, organic meat and fish can sit within the clean eating definition, if prepared freshly and sourced well.

The point is: clean eating is about showing respect for your body. It can be a way for those who have yo-yo dieted to stop calorie counting, then bingeing and then punishing themselves, to take a more positive approach to looking after their bodies.

If you stop obsessively counting calories and studying your bottom in the mirror and instead adopt clean eating as a way to be healthy, you will not only be doing great things for your body but for your mind too.

Traditional diet foods tend to be highly processed and loaded with unhealthy ingredients like sweeteners. Low fat yoghurts and even humous, has added sugar. The list of e numbers on the pack of a diet meal is scary.

Clean eating helps you to nourish your body and your mind, making you feel good about your efforts.

You will need to follow through on your commitment to clean eating but the rewards in terms of how you look and feel will be worth it. Adopting a new eating style is easier if you can find recipes you like.

Certainly with clean eating, you will thrive more quickly if you are prepared to cook a little. No recipe in this book is complicated. I have always hated recipes with inches of ingredients (or centimetres for my European colleagues across the Channel).

Some diets argue that life is made simple by making you live on three juices a day. I have clients who try to do this (before they come to me). Not only is this monotonous and joyless, you risk becoming deficient in important vitamins and minerals, not to mention having no social life.

A word about sugar

While clean eating is the basis of my clinics' programmes, I do think that some versions out there are incredibly high in sugar. If you are concerned about your weight or just your health, tipping a shed load of sugar, whether it's called honey, brown rice syrup or coconut nectar, into your diet is not a good idea.

A high sugar diet puts you at risk of developing Type 2 diabetes and is a risk factor for many other serious health problems including cancer.

But, you say, I thought clean eating was low in sugar. Yes, it's low in processed sugars such as glucose and sucrose, but there are other 'natural' sugars out there from sources such as fruits, dried fruits, honey etc. you need to watch. Why? Because all sugars, natural or not, disrupt your blood sugar and therefore your energy levels, hormone balance and your mood. They also add excess calories, preventing your body getting lean.

I'm not suggesting you never eat an apple again. But I do recommend that you minimise certain 'natural' sugars, in addition to normal sucrose and high frustose corn syrup (which you won't be eating as junk food is off the menu anyway). These extra "natural" sugars to minimise are:

Fructose – from fruit

Maple syrup – has healthy minerals but is still sugar

Brown rice syrup – think of it as syrup dressed up as healthy. Eveything is relative I suppose and compared to golden syrup it is but not on my nutritional programmes.

Coconut sugar/nectar – it may be called "nectar" but it still counts as sugar

Grape juice/apple juice – a common sweetener added to health store snacks.

Dates – most 'healthy' cookies and brownies are sweetened with these. Yes, they have useful minerals, but they are very high in sugar.

Agave syrup – this is a tricky one. It's a syrup processed from cacti. The jury is still out on how this affects your body. It may process in your body like sugar. Some of my clients also find that it affects their mood, just like sugar. So take care with agave. See how you feel emotionally a few hours after eating it. Even if you feel fine, do not go overboard with agave.

Stevia and Xylitol –less of a concern as they are both derived from natural sources and have both been shown not to affect blood sugar but that doesn't mean you can use a ladle with them. Xylitol, if eaten to excess, can also cause stomach discomfort.

I use some fruit, Stevia and agave, but in moderation. Remember there is no such thing as a free lunch, even with a Eating Clean But Keep It Lean lunch. If it tastes sweet it is a source of sugar, however supposedly healthy.

How to eat clean, lean and balanced

My approach is to balance the natural sugars in the clean eating staples of fruits and vegetables. It's really important to include proteins and fats too. Proteins help stabilise your blood sugar, preventing the roller-coaster ride that can cause bingeing. Fats stop your stomach emptying so you feel full.

The easiest way to stay clean but also balanced is to make sure every meal and snack includes carbs, proteins and fats together. If you want to do a juice, add some yoghurt for protein and some Chia seeds for healthy fats. If you're making a salad, boil an egg to go with it and chuck in some walnuts. You get the idea.

Eating Clean But Keep It Lean will not restrict you or make you a freak when you are out and about. It will make you a role model to your friends and family as they see your body transform and your mood and energy lift. There are lots of foods you can eat, even on the go. This book gives you a bit more control of your lunch times as you have recipes for lunches you can eat at home or even use for entertaining plus they are all suitable to be brown bagged for a working lunch. They will ubdoubtedly be better and cheaper than anything that you can buy on the go.

Finally

Don't expect to be perfect. We all have slip-ups. If a cake or a bacon sandwich calls to you, don't tell yourself you're a bad person for succumbing. Just start again at your next meal. Congratulate yourself for your efforts and keep going.

I would be very grateful if you would review this book at the end for me when you are prompted to do so. If you are reading this book on an ereader, you will be prompted to add a review at the end. If you are reading this on PC or tablet, you should get a prompt at the end of this book. If you are reading it in paperback (or listening to this in audio when that format arrives soon!), you can leave a review by visiting the book selling platform where you bought the book. I read all my reviews and your views do matter as I update my books based on reader comment and suggestions.

I would also welcome any suggestions for other subjects you would like covered. You can also reach me by email at hello@threepeaspublishing.com if you head your email FAO Maia Lloyd.

Bonus books

Before we get into the meat of my programme, just to let you know that at the back of this book are two free bonus books to download:

The first is one of my books in this series: Eating Clean But Keep It Lean. It is my book on Sweet Treat foods. You can find download details at the back of this book. In it you will find recipes for desserts: from Chocolate Thins and Berry Frozen Yoghurt to Grilled Pears and Ricotta.

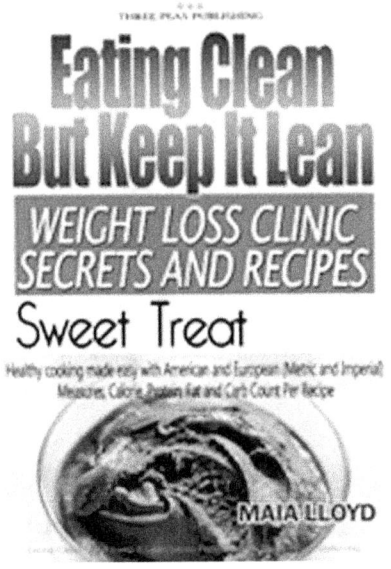

The book also discusses my guidance to my weight loss clients about what makes a dessert Eating Clean But Keep It Lean. Details of how to get this book are at the back of this book with details of all of the books in this Eating Clean But Keep It Lean series.

The other bonus book is from my publishers but it is a good companion to my series. It is called Alcohol Free Drinks and it does what it says on the can, as they say. It probably does a bit more as it is a good mix of celebration drinks, hot toddies, milk shakes, juices and aperitifs.

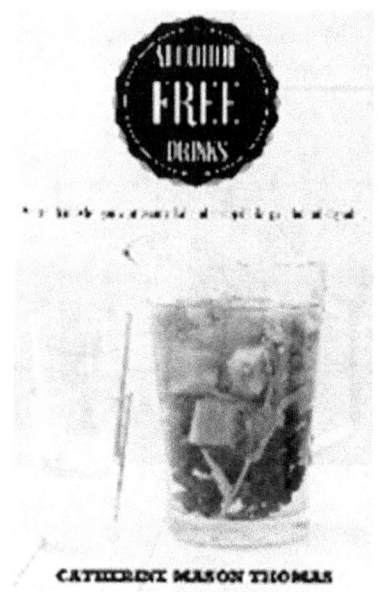

CATHERINE MASON THOMAS

Now on to Chapter 1 and the Salad recipes.

CHAPTER 1
SALADS

Ever eaten one of those sad, shop-bought salads with slightly wilted greens and cold clammy pasta on the bottom? Add a big dollop of greasy dressing and yum! Not.

Eating Clean but Lean salads are filling, healthy and packable, if you want to take them to work.

Tip One: If you are going to transport them, put the wettest ingredients at the bottom of your lunch box and take your dressing separately to prevent wilting.

Top Two: Use a freezer cooler bag to keep everything chilled before you eat it at lunchtime, especially if you do not have access to a fridge. Worst case, refridgerate the ingredients overnight and wrap them in a towel or sweater before you pack them in your bag. The towel or sweater acts as insulation, slowing down the loss of cold, so your food stays fresher and cooler for longer.

Egg Salad with Spicy Tomato Dressing

Eggs are a superfood. Ignore the scare mongering about the yolks. Yes, they have naturally-occurring cholesterol but there is no science to support the idea that this causes cholesterol problems in your body. What egg yolks do have is an amazing concentration of minerals and vitamins, particularly folic acid and choline. Folic acid is a builder vitamin that contributes overall to how healthy you feel.

This recipe is no cook so even the kitchen challenged amongst us can do this one.

Makes: 2 servings

Preparation time: 10 minutes

Cooking time: none

Vegetarian

Ingredients

½ iceberg lettuce 250g/90z, shredded

200g/70z/1 ½ cup frozen sweetcorn, defrosted

2 carrots 150g/5 oz, peeled and grated

1 stick celery/30g/1 ¼ oz, chopped

8 baby plum tomatoes, halved

4 hard boiled eggs, peeled and sliced

2 tablespoons/25g/1oz each fresh, chopped mint and coriander

For the dressing

2 tablespoons/30ml/1 fl oz 0% fat Greek yoghurt

1 teaspoon/5g/1/4oz Stevia-based sweetener

1 tablespoon/15g/1/2oz tomato puree

Splash of Tabasco

Method

Arrange the salad vegetables on two plates. Top with the eggs and sprinkle with the fresh herbs. Put the dressing ingredients in a screw top jar, shake well. Dress just before serving.

Nutritional Content

Makes 2 servings

P/serving

Calories 270

Protein 18g

Carbohydrates 13g

Fat 10g

<u>Jewelled Feta Oomph Salad</u>

The pomegranate in this recipe always reminds me of the Greek myth about the goddess Persephone, who was forced to live for three months a year in the underworld with Hades because she had sucked on pomegranate seeds. This is the Greek mythological explanation for Winter. Pomegranate has always been associated in Asia and Europe with desire…

Another salad with no cooking involved. Just chop and serve or chop and brown bag.

Makes 2 servings

Preparation time: 10 minutes

Cooking time: none

Vegetarian

Ingredients

2 romain or little gem lettuces 250g/9oz, separated into leaves

100g/ 3 ½ oz wild rocket

1 cucumber 400g/14oz, diced

1 red onion 150g/5 oz, thinly sliced

100g/50z feta cheese, cubed

Seeds from half a pomegranate 100g/ 31/2 oz

25g/1 oz walnuts, chopped

For the dressing

2 tablespoons/30ml/1 fl oz of cold-pressed extra virgin olive oil

1 tablespoon/15ml/1/2 fl oz red wine vinegar

1 teaspoon/5g/1/4 oz Stevia-based sweetener

2 tablespoons/20g/3/4 oz chopped dill

Method

Arrange the salad ingredients on two plates.Top with the feta and sprinkle with pomegranate seeds and walnuts. Put the dressing ingredients into a screw topped jar and shake. Dress just before serving.

Nutritional Content

Makes 2 servings

P/serving

Calories 392

Protein 10g

Carbohydrates 12g

Fat 109g

Lean and Clean Chicken Caesar

I love Caesar salad but restaurant versions are very heavy on carb from the croutons and animal fat from the cheese.

This version is lighter because it omits the croutons and decreases the amount of cheese but gives it punch with Dijon mustard.

Anchovies are a fantastic oily fish, so great for decreasing inflammation and calming allergic and reactive symptoms, such as skin rashes and rosacea.

Makes: 2 servings

Preparation time: 10 minutes

Cooking time: none

Serves 2

Ingredients

1 head cos lettuce 250g/9oz, broken into leaves

12 cherry tomatoes

200g/ 7oz cooked, skinless chicken breast, sliced

2 tablespoons pumpkin seeds, toasted in a hot pan and cooled.

For the dressing

1 egg yolk

4 anchovies, drained on kitchen paper

1 clove garlic, crushed

½ lemon, juice only

1 teaspoon Dijon mustard

25g parmesan cheese, grated

1 tablespoon cold-press extra virgin olive oil

1 tablespoon white wine vinegar

Pepper

Method:

Arrange the lettuce and tomatoes on two plates. Top with the chicken. Put the dressing ingredients into a food processor and process till smooth. Dress just before serving. Sprinkle over the toasted pumpkin seeds.

Nutritional Content

Makes 2 servings

P/serving

Calories 381

Protein 45g

Carbohydrates 6g

Fat 18g

You can make a really good hot version of this by cooking the chicken breast from raw: bash the chicken breast out so it is no more than 2cm think, sprinkle it with smoked paprika or cayenne, dry fry it for five minutes on each side, let it sit covered for 5 minutes, then slice and serve with the salad. The nutritional values, including the calorie count, are the same.

Chinese Chicken, Green Mango and Mint Salad

The mint and mango in this dish really zing your cells. The mint is also a digestive so you will feel very lean the next day, no bloating.

If you choose the hot version explained at the bottom of the recipe, this is also a nice salad to serve for guests or as a light supper.

Makes: 2 servings

Preperation time: 10 minutes

Cooking time: none

Ingredients

2 little gem lettuces 200g/70z separated into leaves

1 cucumber 400g/14 oz, sliced

2 carrots 150g/60z, peeled and grated

240g/8 ½ oz skinless chicken breast, sliced

1 green mango, peeled and cut into matchsticks

For the dressing

Juice of 2 limes

1 small red chilli, deseeded and finely chopped

2 tablespoons/30ml/1 ¾ fl oz fish sauce

1 tablespoon/15g/1/2 oz Stevia-based sweetener

1 teaspoon/5 ml/1/4 fl oz sesame oil

2 shallots, finely chopped.

Method

Arrange the salad ingredients on two plates. Top with chicken and mango. Put the dressing ingredients in a screw topped jar and shake. Dress just before serving. N.B. This dressing tastes better if you let the flavour develop over 4 hours or more.

Nutritional Content

Makes 2 servings

P/serving

Calories 330

Protein 32g

Carbohydrate 49g

Fat 6g

You can make a really good hot version of this by cooking the chicken breast from raw: bash the chicken breast out so it is no more than 2cm think, sprinkle it with Chinese 5 Spice powder, dry fry it for five minutes on each side, let it sit covered for 5 minutes, then slice and serve with the salad. The nutritional values, including the calorie count, are the same.

Turkey and Broccoli Salad with Gremolata

Sounds posh. Gremolata simply means a herby, citrously dressing.

Turkey contains tryptophan which is a precursor to serotonin, the happy hormone. It helps to keep you calm and centred.

Broccoli is the king of detox foods so it helps your body, particularly your liver, get rid of toxins. The result – better skin in particular.

Makes: 2 servings

Preparation time: 10 mimutes

Cooking time: none

Ingredients

225/8 oz broccxoli florets steamed and allowed to cool

1 hearts of romaine lettuce 250g/70z, leaves separated

100g/3 ½ oz watercress

8 black olives, pitted and chopped

240g/8 ½ oz skinless cooked turkey breast, sliced

Pinch of chilli flakes

For the Gremolata

1 garlic clove, peeled

Zest and juice of 1 lemon

Bunch each of parsley and rocket

2 tablespoons/30ml/1 fl oz cold-pressed extra virgin olive oil

Method

Arrange the salad ingredients on two plates. Top with the turkey and sprinkle with chilli flakes. Put the dressing ingredients in a food processor and pulse to create a sauce. Dress just before serving.

Nutritional Content

Makes 2 servings

P/serving

Calories 339

Protein 36g

Carbohydrates 6g

Fat 19g

Salmon and Avocado Salad With Wasabi Vinaigrette

Salads with fresh salmon are very fashionable girl lunch food but they are also very clean and lean. Yes, salmon is an oily fish but the oil is high in Omega 3 fatty acids which are needed by your body in virtually every function, from building cell walls to hormone production. Avocado is also rich in Omega 3 and also in lots of minerals, including copper.

The dressing is astringent to cut the richness of the fish and the avocado.

Keep the dressing separate until just before you serve the salad. If you're packing this one, put the avocado in with the dressing to stop it turning brown.

I think cooked salmon is nice cold so this works well as a brown bag lunch.

Makes 2 servings

Preparation time: 10 minutes

Cooking time: none

<u>Ingredients</u>

2 heads red chicory, separated into leaves

2 handfuls baby spinach leaves

12 baby tomatoes

2 x 120g filet of cooked salmon

1 large, ripe avocado, peeled, stoned and sliced.

<u>For the dressing</u>

2 limes, juice only

2 tablespoons/30ml1 ½ fl oz cold-pressed extra virgin olive oil

2 teaspoon/10g/1/4 oz wasabi

1 teaspoon/5g/1/4 oz agave syrup

<u>Method</u>

Arrange the salad ingredients on two plates. Top with the salmon and avocado. Put the dressing ingredients into a screw topped jar and shake gently. Dress just before serving.

Nutritional Content

Makes 2 servings

P/serving

Calories 393

Protein 25g

Carbohydrates 18g

Fat 28g

Kicking Mackerel Salad

Smoked mackerel is oily fish so you get your Omega 3s. The horseradish intensifies the flavour so this one will definitely wake you up if you are flagging at lunchtime.

Makes: 2 servings

Preparation: 10 minutes

Cooking: none

Ingredients

1 cos lettuce 250g/3 ½ oz, separated into leaves

2 sticks celery 60g/2 ½ oz, chopped

1 red onion 150g/5 oz, sliced thinly

1 x 120g filet of smoked mackerel, skin removed, but into two pieces.

For the Horseradish Dressing

4 tablespoons/60ml/2 1/2 fl oz/1/4 cup 0% fat Greek yoghurt

1 teaspoon/5g/1/4 oz Stevia-based sweetener

2 teaspoons/10g/1/4 oz creamed horseradish (from a jar)

Squeeze of lemon juice

Method

Arrange the salad on two plates. Top with the mackerel. Mix together the dressing ingredients. Dress just before serving.

Nutritional Content

Makes 2 servings

P/serv

Calories 421

Protein 24g

Carbohydrate 7g

Fat 32g

Asian Slaw With Prawns

This recipe is a good combination of the classic coleslaw ingredients and Asian flavours – ginger and sesame. Instead of heavy mayonaise, you have a Chinese style dressing. This one really improves if you leave it in the fridge overnight, or you can make a big batch and keep it for up to five days in the fridge in an airtight container.

Makes: 2 servings

Perparation time: 10 minutes

Cooking: none

Ingredients

½ head white cabbage 400g/14oz, shredded

½ head red cabbage, 400g/140z peeled and grated

100g/ 3 ½ oz radishes, finely sliced

200g/7 0z/ 2 cups beansprouts

240g/7 ½ oz cooked prawns

2 tablespoons/30g/1 ¼ oz chopped almonds or brazil nuts

2 tablespoons/20g/3/4 oz chopped coriander leaves

For the dressing:

Zest and juice of 1 lime

2 teaspoons/10g/1/4 oz Stevia-based sweetener

2 teaspoons/10g/1/4 fl oz sesame oil

½ red chilli, deseeded and chopped

2cm piece of fresh ginger, peeled and grated

Method

Arrange the salad ingredients on two plates. Top with the prawns and sprinkle on the peanuts (or almonds or brazils, if you prefer) and coriander. Put the dressing ingredients in a screw topped jar and shake. Dress just before serving.

Nutritional Content

Makes 2 servings

p/serving

Calories 346

Protein 30g

Carbohydrates 8g

Fat 13g

CHAPTER 2
SOUPS

You can spend a lot of money on shop bought soups. Now, they are better than the alternative, carb-heavy sandwiches and flacid, oily salads but if you make you own, you save money and ensure that they are the are clean and lean.

Soup is a great lunch or light dinner idea. If you make it in advance, it's ready, quick. Just reheat in a pan or microwave for three or four minutes and you're ready to go. Plus it packs really well in a flask . And it is a great way to get your five-a-day.

One important point about my Eating Clean But Keep It Lean soups is they all contain protein. This is key to balancing your blood sugar and getting lean. A vegetable soup breaks down into sugar in the body. For soups based on root veggies such as butternut squash or carrot, that's quite a lot of sugar. As we know, the body stores excess sugar as fat. So that apparently healthy carrot or sweet potato soup can actually be quite fattening.

Add some Clean Eating protein such as chicken, tuna, prawns, beans, eggs or tofu and the soup immediately becomes more balanced. Your blood sugar is stabilised and you won't be starving again a couple of hours later.

Soup is especially important for reducing hunger because research says that it pushes down appetite-stimulating grehlin levels. For example if you eat chicken and a glass of water, the water passes straight through the stomach. But if you eat chicken soup, the water in the soup stays in the stomach, adding volume and switching off grehlin.

My soups are filling and satisfying, so give them a try.

Soups work best when you make a big batch, so I've done these recipes for four. You can eat one portion then chill or freeze the rest.

Courgette and White Bean Soup

Beans are great as they release their carohydrate slowly and they contain insoluble fibre so they keep you full and keep your digestive tract clean. An internal spring clean!

Makes: 4 servings

Preparation: 5 minutes

Cooking: 35 minutes

vegetarian

Ingredients

Spray oil (or make your own with cold-pressed olive, hemp or coconut oil in an old oil spray bottle)

1 onion 200g/7 oz, chopped

1/2 leek 75g/3 oz, halved, sliced and soaked in cold water

1 clove garlic, crushed

2 courgettes 350g/12 oz, cut lengthways, seeds removed, diced

300g/11oz/1 1/4 cups dried haricot beans.

Handful of parsley, chopped

1 litre/1 ¾ pints/4 cups vegetable stock

100ml/3 ½ fl oz/ ½ cup skimmed milk

Salt and white pepper

Method

Spritz a saucepan with spray oil and gently fry the onion for 3 -4 minutes, then add the the garlic and cook for 1 minute. Add the rest of the ingredients except the parsley. Bring up to the boil then turn down to a simmer and cook for 20-25 minutes until the beans are tender. Add the parsley, season and serve.

You can blend this soup if you like your soups smooth. This one becomes velvety if you blend it.

Nutritional Content

Makes 4 servings

p/serving

Calories 340

Protein 33g

Carbohydrates 49g

Fat 3g

Edamame and Basil Soup

This soup is very fresh looking with its bright green colour. The basil gives it depth and the edamame (soy beans in old English) provide the protein. The basil also give this soup a nutritional punch as herbs are particular rich in vitamins.

Makes: 4 servings

Preparation: 2 minutes

Cooking 15 minutes

Vegetarian

Ingredients

200g/7 oz/4 cups frozen edamame beans

200g/7 oz/ 4 cups frozen peas

1 litre/1 ¾ pints/4 cups hot vegetable stock

6 spring onions, chopped

1 large bunch fresh basil leaves

100g/ 3 ½ oz rocket leaves

200ml/7 fl oz/ 3/4 cup skimmed milk or soy or almond milk

Method

Put the edamame beans, peas and stock in a saucepan, bring up to the boil and the simmer for 5 minutes. Stir in the rest of the ingredients and cook for another 5 minutes. Take off the heat to cool slightly. Transfer half the mixture to a bowl and use a hand blender to process till smooth. Add back into the chunky mixture, put back on the heat to bring back up to the boil and serve.

Nutritional Content

Makes 4 servings

P/serving

Calories 240

Protein 11g

Carbohydrates 11g

Fat 3g

Tuscan Tomato Soup

I love fresh tomato soup but I am never going to stand there and peel tomato skins. This soup uses canned, chopped tomatoes so you get the taste without the labour. Tomatoes contain a nutrient called Lycopene which is only activated by heating so this is one vegetable (technically it is a fruit) that is better for you cooked.

Makes 4 servings

Preparation: 10 minutes

Cooking: 40 minutes

Vegetarian

<u>Ingredients</u>

Spray olive oil (or make you own – see Courgette Soup recipe)

1 small red onion 150g/5oz, finely chopped

1 clove garlic, crushed

1 carrot 75g/3 oz, peeled and diced

2 sticks celery 60g/2 ½ oz, chopped

400g/14oz/2 cups chopped tomatoes

400g/14oz/2 cups canned mixed beans, drained

1 tablespoon/25g/1/2 oz tomato paste

800ml/1 ¼ pints/3 ½ cups vegetable stock

2 sprigs fresh thyme

Salt and pepper

<u>Method</u>

Spritz a non stick saucepan with cooking spray and fry the onion for 3 – 4 minutes till soft. Add the garlic, carrot, and celery and cook for 5 more minutes. Add more stock if starts to stick. Add the rest of the ingredients, bring up to the boil, then simmer with a lid on for 20 – 30 minutes until the vegetables are cooked. Take off the heat and allow to cool slightly. Transfer half the mixture to a bowl and use a hand blender to process till smooth. Add back into the chunky mixture and put back on the heat. Bring up to the boil and serve.

Nutritional Content

Makes 4 servings

P/serving

Calories 172

Protein 8g

Carbohydrates 22g

Fat 5g

Moroccan Broad Bean Soup

This is an interesting, spicy soup. The Harissa gives it a middle eastern flavour. Harissa is a spicy paste you get in a jar. If you can't get it, use flaked chilli but add it gradually as that stuff packs a heat punch.

Makes 4 servings

Preparation: 5 minutes

Cooking: 20 minutes

Vegetarian

Ingredients:

Spray olive oil (or make your own – see Courgette Soup recipe)

1 onion 200g/7 oz, chopped

1 clove garlic, crushed

2 celery sticks 60g/ 2 ½ oz chopped

2 teaspoons/10g/ ¼ oz ground cumin

1 teaspoon/ 5g/ ¼ oz harissa paste

1 litre/1 ¾ pints/4 ½ cups vegetable stock

400g/14 oz/ 2 cups canned chopped tomatoes

400g/14 oz/ 2 cups frozen broad beans

Zest and juice of 1 lemon

Salt and pepper

1 large handful each fresh coriander and parsley leaves

Method

Spritz a non stick saucepan with spray oil and fry the onion and celery for 3 – 4 minutes. Add the garlic, cumin and Harissa and fry for 1 minute (add a splash of water if it starts to stick). Add the stock, tomatoes and broad beans, bring up to the boil and simmer with a lid on for 10 minutes. Add the lemon, season and take off the heat. Transfer half the mixture to a bowl and use a hand blender to process till smooth. Add back into the chunky mixture, put back on the heat, bring back up to the boil and serve.

Nutritional Content

Makes 4 servings

P/serving

Calories 116

Protein 31g

Carbohydrates 64g

Fat 4g

Spicy Lentil Soup

Lentils are one of my favourites for sustained energy. This version is similar to dhal in that it is Indian spiced. This keeps well in the fridge.

You can also use this as a dip with julienne vegatables if you use less vegetable stock. Then serve it 50:50 on a plate with 0% fat Greek yoghurt and raw stick (julienne) vegetables.

Makes 4 servings

Preparation: 5 minutes

Cooking: 40 minutes

Vegetarian

Ingredients

Spray olive oil (or make your own – see recipe for Courgette Soup)

1 onion 200g/7 oz, chopped

1 clove garlic, peeled and chopped

1 teaspoon/ 5g/ ¼ oz each ground ginger and garam masala

1 litre/ 1 ¾ pints/4 ½ cups vegetable stock

1 carrot 75g/3 oz and 1 parsnip 75g/ 3oz, chopped

1 lemon, cut in half

160g/5 ¼ oz/2/3 cup dried puy lentils

Salt and pepper

4 tablespoons/60ml/1/2 cup 0% fat Greek yoghurt

Method

Spritz a non stick saucepan with spray oil, add the onion and cook for 3 - 4 minutes to soften. Add the garlic and fry for 1 minute, then add the spices and cook for another minute. Pour in the stock, vegetables, lemon and lentils. Bring up to the boil, then simmer with a lid on for 25 – 30 minutes until the lentils are soft. Remove from the heat and allow to cool slightly. Remove the lemon. Use a hand blender to process till smooth. Season, stir in the yoghurt and serve.

Nutritional Content

Makes 4 servings

P/serving

Calories 255

Protein 11g

Carbohydrates 30g

Fat 5g

Mexican Pinto Bean Soup With Avocado Salsa

I have always loved Pinto bean soup. Back before the explosion of Southern American/Mexican fast healthy food in London (think of the Wahaca chain), the only place you could get really good pinto bean soup was US restaurant and pre-theatre institution, Joe Allen. That was a fantastic soup and here is my version.

This version with Avocado will have your work colleagues wanting to try it. It is also interesting enough for a dinner party first course or an informal, friends supper.

Makes 4 servings

Preparation: 10 minutes

Cooking: 55 minutes

Vegetarian

Ingredients:

Spray olive oil (or make your own – see recipe for Courgette Soup)

1 onion 200g/7 oz, chopped

6 cloves garlic, crushed

1 fresh red chilli, deseeded and chopped

1 red and 1 yellow pepper, 350g/12 oz deseeded and roughly chopped

1 teaspoon/ 5g/ ¼ oz each cayenne pepper, cumin, coriander and smoked paprika

2 tablespoons/30ml/ 1 fl oz tomato puree

400g/14 oz/2 cups canmed pinto or red kidney beans, drained

800g/28oz/4 cups canned chopped tomatoes

400ml/14 fl oz/1 ¾ cups vegetable stock

2 tablespoons/ 30ml/1 fl oz red wine vinegar

1 tablespoon/ 15g/1/2 oz Stevia-based sweetener

Salt and pepper

For the avocado salsa

1 ripe avocado 170g/6 oz, peeled, stoned and diced

½ red onion/100g/ 3 ½ oz, finely sliced

½ red chilli, deseeded and finely sliced

1 tablespoon/ 15g/1/2 oz fresh, chopped coriander leaves

1 lime, juice only

1 tablespoon/15ml cold pressed extra virgin olive oil

Pinch of salt.

Method

Spritz a non stick saucepan with spray oil and fry the onion for 3 – 4 minutes till soft. Add the garlic, chilli, spices and red and yellow peppers and cook for 5 minutes, adding a splash of water if it starts to stick. Add the red wine vinegar, sweetener and tomato puree and cook for 5 minutes. Then add the beans, chopped tomatoes and vegetable stock. Season and bring up to the boil, cover and simmer for 30 – 40 minutes. To make the avocado salsa, mix all the ingredients together. Serve the soup with a dollop of the salsa on top.

Nutritional Content

Makes 4 servings

P/serving

Calories 281

Protein 11g

Carbohydrates 33g

Fat 14g

Miso Soup with Butternut Squash and Tofu

This recipe is a pretty genuine Miso soup. If you do not have the time or availability of ingredients, you can use a good Miso instant soup and just add the tofu and vegetables. However, if you want to have a go, find a local Japanese deli or order ingredients online.

Makes: 4 servings

Preparation: 1 hour 10 minutes to make the dashi

Cooking: 25 minutes

Vegetarian

Ingredients for the dashi

6g piece of dried kombu (Japanese seaweed)

2 tablespoons/1.5g dried bonito flakes

1.25 litres/ 2 pints/ 5 cups water

Ingredients for the soup

500g/ 1 lb 2 oz butternut squash, skin on, cut into chunks

225g/8oz broccoli cut into small florets

425g/ 15 oz tofu, drained and cubed

Method

To make the dashi

Soak the kombu in a saucepan with the water for 1 hour. Bring the water up to the boil, removing the kombu just before it reaches the boil. Add the bonito flakes and simmer gently for 5 minutes. Switch off the heat and allow to stand for 5 minutes before pouring through a sieve.

To make the soup, put the butternut squash in a steamer and steam for 15 minutes till tender. Turn off the heat and allow to cool in the steamer. Cook the mangetout in boiling water for 2 minutes till cooked but still a little crunchy, plunge into cold water. Set aside. Scoop out the butternut squash flesh from the peel and put in a food processor. Process till you get a smooth puree. Add the miso and mix well. Heat the dashi in a saucepan and gradually stir in the butternut squash, bringing up to a gentle simmer. Add the tofu, heat through and serve.

Nutritional Content

Makes 4 servings

P/serving

Calories 123

Protein 25g

Carbohydrates 3g

Fat 5g

Thai Chicken and Mushroom Broth

A simple Thai soup with a good red curry flavour. You can bulk this up so you could use whatever green vegatables you have in the fridge, so broccoli, courgettes, leaks, cabbage or kale. See what you can find. Adding the vegatables will not alter the nutritional calculations provided you stick to green vegeatables (not peas – too much sugar).

Makes: 4 servings

Preparation: 5 minutes

Cooking: 10 minutes

Ingredients

1 litre/1 ¾ pints/ 4 ½ cups hot chicken stock

1 tablespoon/ 15g/1/2 oz Thai red curry paste

1 tablespoon/15ml fish sauce

2 teaspoons/10g/ ¼ oz Stevia-based sweetener

Zest and juice of 2 limes

100g/3 1/2oz Portobello mushrooms, sliced

Bunch of spring onions sliced, white and greens separated

400g/14 oz cooked, skinless chicken breast, cubed

Method

Put everything apart from the green part of the spring onions into a saucepan. Bring up to a boil, put a lid on and simmer for 5 minutes. Add the chicken and cook for 3 more minutes. Serve topped with the spring onion greens.

Nutritional Content

P/serving Makes 4 servings

Calories 123

Protein 25g

Carboydrates 3g

Fat 5g

Chinese Pork and Spinach Broth

Makes 4 servings

Preparation: 5 minutes

Cooking: 8 minutes

Ingredients

400g/14 oz pork tenderloins, cut into thin strips

1 litre/1 ¾ pints/4 ½ cups chicken stock

2 tablespoon/ 15ml/1/2 fl oz soy sauce

2 teaspoons/ 10ml Chinese 5 spice powder

4cm piece of ginger, peeled and cut into matchsticks

500g/1 lb 2 oz oz baby spinach

1 red chilli, deseeded and chopped

Bunch spring onions, sliced

Method

Put everything into a large saucepan, put a lid on and simmer gently for 8 minutes till the pork is cooked. Serve.

Nutritional Content

Makes 4 servings

P/serving

Calories 168

Protein 23g

Carbohydrates 4g

Fat 10g

Quillade (French "kill-ard" – ham and harocot bean soup)

The English have their version – ham and split pea soup. The French equivalent is this ham and haricot bean soup. Try to avoid using any smoked meat as it is just too salty.

This is very simple and hearty soup and high in protein. You can "pimp" this soup with herbs - bay and sage or leave it this simple.

If I am feeling at all in need of vitamins, I make this soup and increase by a factor of three, the amount of kale in the soup. You could also use spinach or watercress instead.

Makes 4 servings

Preparation: 10 minutes

Cooking: 1 hr 20 mins

Ingredients

400g/14 oz unsmoked ham hock

1 litre/1 ¾ pints/ 4 ½ cups cold water

125g/4 oz/ 2/3 cup dried haricot beans, soaked overnight and drained

500ml/3/4 pint/2 cups water

Olive oil cooking spray (or make your own – see recipe for Edamame Soup)

1 onion 200g/7oz, chopped

2 carrots 150g/50z, peeled and chopped

75g/ 3oz turnip or swede, peeled and diced

125g/4 oz curly kale, chopped

2 cloves garlic, finely chopped

1 tablespoon, 10g/1/4 oz chopped fresh parsley

Method

Put the ham hock into a saucepan and cover with the water. Bring up to the boil, cover and simmer for 45 minutes, turning it over as the liquid reduces. The meat should be falling off the bone. Leave to cool in the water, then lift out the ham and set aside. Pour the liquid from the ham through a sieve and reserve the liquid. Meanwhile, put the beans in another saucepan with 500ml water. Bring up to the boil then cover and simmer for 45 minutes, removing any scum that comes up to the surface with a spoon. Drain and set aside. Spritz a non stick saucepan with cooking spray and fry the onion for 3 – 4 minutes. Add the carrots and cook for 5 – 10 minutes till soft, adding some of the ham stock if it starts to stick. Add 1 litre of ham stock , the turnip/swede and simmer for 10 minutes. Meanwhile, remove the skin from the ham. Tear the meat into small pieces. Add this, plus the kale and beans to the soup and simmer for 5 minutes. Remove the pan from the heat, stir in the garlic, parsley and black pepper and serve.

Nutritional Content

Makes: 4 servings

P/serving

Calories 382

Protein 39g

Carbohydrates 33g

Fat 6g

Hungarian Beef and Beetroot Soup

I got this recipe from a Hungarian family living in London. I have lightened it slightly. My Hungarian friends were living in a very small bedsit with a shared kitchen and they had invited me to supper. They made this one pot meal and we all sat around in their bedroom to eat it. They also offered me slices of cured pork fat, which were more of a culture shock. A really memorable night for the food and the stories.

Makes: 4 servings

Preparation: 20 minutes

Cooking: 1 hr 40 mins

Ingredients

Olive oil cooking spray (or make you own – see recipe for Courgette Soup)

400g/14 oz stewing steak, cut into small dice

1 onion 200g/7 oz, chopped

2 cloves of garlic, crushed

1 tablespoons/30g/1 ¼ oz paprika

1 teaspoon/5g cumin seeds

250g/9 oz potatoes, peeled and diced

400g/14 oz/2 cups canned chopped tomatoes

750ml/1 ¼ pints/2 ½ cups beef stock

2 fresh beetroot 500g/1 lb 2 oz, scrubbed and trimmed

1 tablespoon/10g chopped dill

2 tablespoons/20g chopped parsley.

Method

Preheat the oven to 200/gas mark 6. Spritz a non stick saucepan with cooking spray. Fry the beef in batches to brown and set aside. Spritz the pan again and add the onion. Fry for 3 – 4 minutes to soften, then add the garlic and spices. Cook for 1 minute, adding a splash of stock if it starts to stick. Add the potatoes and coat with the onion/garlic/spice mixture. Put the beef back in, as well as the chopped tomatoes and stock. Season, cover and simmer very gently for 1 ½ hours till the beef is tender. Meanwhile, wrap the beetroot in foil and bake for 40 minutes. Take out of the oven, allow to cool then peel and cut into 1 cm dice. Add to the soup, sprinkle with the herbs and serve.

Nutritional Content

Makes 4 servings

Calories 383

Protein 39g

Carbohydrates 28g

Fat 11g

Spanish Fish Soup

Fish is a great choice for any meal because fish, like turkey, contains tryptophan which our bodies use to make seretonin, the happy hormone. The satisfaction in this soup comes from the addition of potatoes and chick peas to give the soup bulk and texture.

Serves 4

Makes: 4 servings

Preparation: 10 minutes

Cooking: 30 minutes

Ingredients

Olive oil cooking spray (or make your own – see recipe for Edamame Soup)

1 onion 200g/7 oz, chopped

2 garlic cloves, crushed

1 teaspoon/5g each paprika and cayenne pepper

Zest and juice of 1 lemon

400g/14 oz/2 cups canned chopped tomatoes

600ml/ 1 pint/ 2 ½ cups vegetable stock

250g/9 oz potatoes, peeled and cut into small cubes

400g/14 oz/ 2 cups canned chickpeas, drained

500g/1 lb 2 oz firm white fish such as cod or pollock, cut into large chunks.

Salt and pepper

Handful of fresh parsely, chopped

Method

Spritz a non stick saucepan with spray oil and fry the onion for 3 – 4 minutes till soft. Add the garlic and spices and fry for another minute. Add the potatoes, coat with the garlic/onion/spice mixture then add the lemon juice and zest and allow to sizzle for 30 seconds. Add the tomatoes, stock, season and bring up to the boil. Put a lid on and simmer for 10 – 15 minutes till the poatoes are almost cooked, then add the chickpeas and fish and cook for 8 minutes till the fish is cooked. Sprinkle with parsley and serve.

Nutritional Content

Makes: 4 servings

Calories: 298

Protein: 32g

Carbohydrates: 34g

Fat 5g

Healthy Prawn Laksa

I have kept the carb count down in this soup by using bean sprouts in place of the glass noodles usually found in a laksa. You still get all the flavour from the coconut milk and the red curry paste.

Makes 4 servings

Preparation: 15 minutes

Cooking: 10 minutes

Ingredients

Olive oil cooking spray (or make your own – see recipe for Courgette Soup)

1 tablespoon/15g/1/2 oz Thai red curry paste

750 ml/1 ¼ pints/2 ¾ cups vegetable stock

400g/ 14 oz prawns, shells removed and cleaned and de-veined

1 red pepper 175g/6 oz, deseeded and sliced

600g/1lb 5 oz/6 cups beansprouts

400ml/ 14 oz/ 2 cups reduced fat coconut milk

Juice of 1 lime

2 tablespoons/ 15g/1/2 oz Stevia based sweetener

Small handful chopped coriander leaves.

Method

Spritz a non stick saucepan with cooking spray and fry the curry paste for 1 – 2 minutes, add the stock, bring up to the boil and then add the prawns. Cover and simmer for 5 minutes till they are pink and cooked. Add the pepper and beansprouts and cook for 2 minutes, then the coconut milk. Bring back up to a simmer, add the lime juice and sweetener and serve.

Nutritional Content

Makes: 4 servings

Calories 203

Protein 27g

Carbohydrates 10g

Fat 15g

CONCLUSION

The legal bit is next and then I have some concluding thoughts about weight loss, details of how to download my free, bonus books and also news of the rest of my series: **Eating Clean But Keep It Lean**.

So, you are now armed with lots of Eating Clean But Keep It Lean Eating choices for your lunches.

I hope you will be convinced that eating in this healthful way is neither bland nor boring.

The results for the way forward in terms of how you feel and look outweigh any perceived "convenience" of grabbing a sandwich or worse, on the hoof. Longer term by choosing to eat simply and naturally, you are paying into a personal vault for your health. The steps you take now to take charge of your nutrition will mean that you age more slowly and the degenerative and purely preventable, diet-related diseases of Type 2 diabetes and hypertension should never happen to you. Other deseases we know now have a lifestyle component: cancer and dementia, are much less likely to happen to you, just because you give your body a chance to operate optimally. Those conditions whose symptoms are exacerbated by poor diet choices: arthritis, exzema, asthma, IBS and PCOS, you can choose to live with the least severe symptoms.

I know this because I see the reversal of some diseases and improvement in symptoms of others, once my programmes have kicked in.

So if you want to dodge the bullet of some diseases altogether and for others, give yourself the best chance of avoiding them or having them at their least severe, the choice you make now to eat well, is the wisest, absolutely wisest investment you can make in yourself.

My twist on clean eating, is to make sure that this includes lean. This also has undeniably positive health effects. Much has been said about how being overweight is more healthy than being overweight. I am afraid that this is just not supported by the science. Carrying excess fat has direct effect on your chances of contracting cancer, and for the worse. That is because, certainly for women, excess fat is a factory for oestrogen. Oestrogen is a growth hormone which helps cancer cells to multiply. If you are unconvinced about the effect of oestogen, just look at the correlation between overweight in young girls and the early onset of puberty, that is excess oestrogen at work.

Excess weight also puts strain on your joints, exacerbating arthritis and the pain that comes from sore joints.

But there is also a question here of how you want to live your life. Excess weight closes down your options. For example, I ride horses. Beyond a certain weight, you won't find a horse to ride.

So, my programme is also an opportunity to take control of your weight in a long term sustainable way so you never have to expect to become overweight as you age.

There is no law that says that over 40 or 50, you need to become fat and immobile. If you are going that way, well done for reading this book and get on with opening up your options again by reclaiming our health and vitality.

If you are already Eating Clean But Keep It Lean, I hope the food in this book adds to your repertoire and you find some firm favourites in here.

If you enjoyed this book, this is part of a whole series I have written to publish my recipes from my weight loss clinics. One of these books, the Sweet Treat recipe book, is free as part of my bonus books (see below), the others are my nutritional plans focussed on real food eaten everyday and are available from Amazon.

Each book has lots of recipes from my clinics, ones that have worked with my clients to help them lose weight. The introduction to each book also tells a little of the story of my approach at my clinics so you understand what foods are best for weight loss.

You can find the complete series, book by book, at Amazon and they are also listed below. Get the set or start off with a couple of books to inspire you and inform you about the Eating Clean But Keep it Lean approach to particular meals, say Dinner and Brown Bag Lunches, for example.

If you have comments or questions, you can also get in contact with me by emailing me at hello@threepeaspublishing.com

Here is the complete series. You can buy single books or the whole series.

Just search "Maia Lloyd Author Page" on Amazon

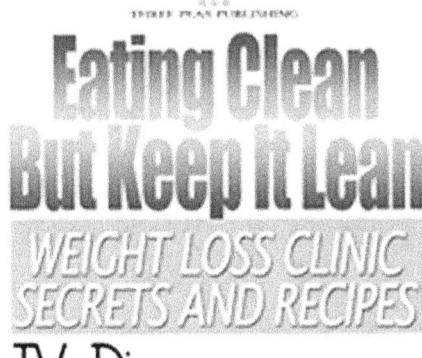

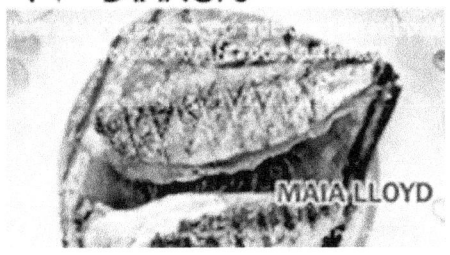

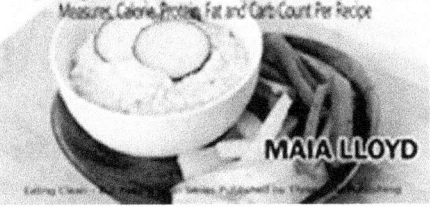

✳ ✳ ✳
THREE PEAS PUBLISHING

Eating Clean
But Keep It Lean

WEIGHT LOSS CLINIC
SECRETS AND RECIPES

Soups & Salads

Healthy cooking made easy with American and European (Metric and Imperial)
Measures Calorie, Protein, Fat and Carb Count Per Recipe

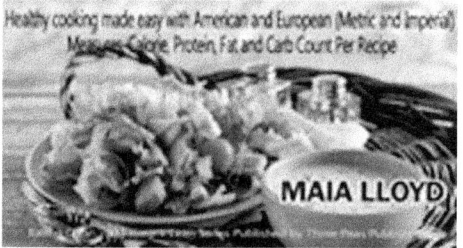

MAIA LLOYD

✳ ✳ ✳
THREE PEAS PUBLISHING

Eating Clean
But Keep It Lean

WEIGHT LOSS CLINIC
SECRETS AND RECIPES

Brown Bag Lunches

Healthy cooking made easy with American and European (Metric and Imperial)
Measures, Calorie, Protein, Fat and Carb Count Per Recipe

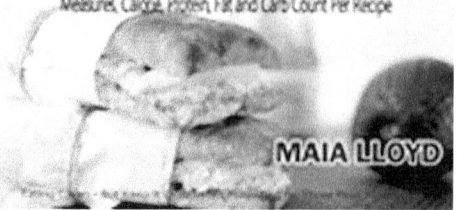

MAIA LLOYD

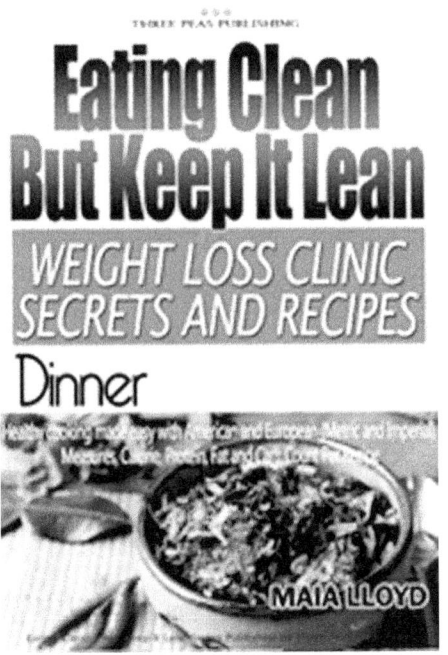

Bonus books

The first is one of my books in this series: Eating Clean But Keep It Lean. It is my book on Sweet Treat foods. In it you will find recipes for desserts: from Chocolate Thins and Berry Frozen Yoghurt to Grilled Pears and Ricotta.

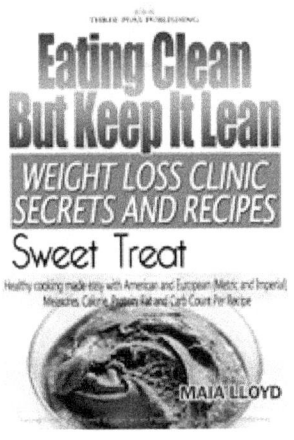

The book also discusses my guidance to my weight loss clients about what makes a dessert Eating Clean But Keep It Lean. Details of how to get this book are at the back of this book with details of all of the books in this Eating Clean But Keep It Lean series.

You can download this at: www.threepeaspublishing.com/eatingcleanbutkeepitleans weettreat

The other bonus book is from my publishers but it is a good companion to my series. It is called Alcohol Free Drinks and it does what it says on the can, as they say. It probably does a bit more as it is a good mix of celebration drinks, hot toddies, milk shakes, juices and aperitifs.

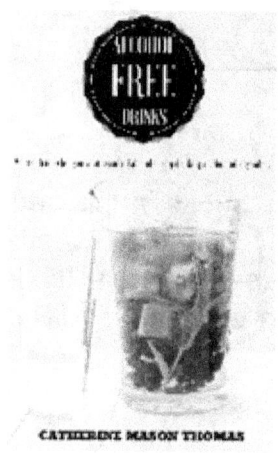

You can download this at: www.threepeaspublishing.com/alcoholfreedrinks

If you are interested in nutrition, fitness and wellness, you can subscribe to news, offers and How To videos on nutrition (including my books), nutrition and resilience via my publisher, Three Peas Publishing. To subscribe, go to www.threepeaspublishing.com. Three Peas Media also has a YouTube Channel "Three Peas Media" which provides videos on fitness and nutrition and resilience.

Finally, I would be very grateful if you would review this book for me when you are prompted to do so if you are reading this book on an ereader, or by visiting the book selling platform if you are reading this in paperback. I read all my reviews and I would also welcome and suggestions for other ubjects you would like covered. You can also reach me by email at hello@threepeaspublishing.com if you head your email FAO Maia Lloyd.

Good luck and value your health.

With best wishes

Maia Lloyd

www.ingramcontent.com/pod-product-compliance
Lightning Source LLC
Chambersburg PA
CBHW071127280526
45787CB00003B/1197